Teaching Transcultural Care

Books

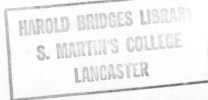

0412440806

Teaching Transcultural Care

A guide for teachers of nursing and health care

Paula McGee

Principal Lecturer at the Nursing Research Unit,
Birmingham Polytechnic

CHAPMAN & HALL

London · Glasgow · New York · Tokyo · Melbourne · Madras

Published by Chapman & Hall, 2–6 Boundary Row, London SE1 8HN

Chapman & Hall, 2–6 Boundary Row, London SE1 8HN, UK

Blackie Academic & Professional, Wester Cleddens Road, Bishopbriggs, Glasgow G64 2NZ, UK

Chapman & Hall, 29 West 35th Street, New York NY10001, USA

Chapman & Hall Japan, Thomson Publishing Japan, Hirakawacho Nemoto Building, 6F, 1–7–11 Hirakawa-cho, Chiyoda-ku, Tokyo 102, Japan

Chapman & Hall Australia, Thomas Nelson Australia, 102 Dodds Street, South Melbourne, Victoria 3205, Australia

Chapman & Hall India, R. Seshadri, 32 Second Main Road, CIT East, Madras 600 035, India

Distributed in the USA and Canada by Singular Publishing Group, Inc., 4284 41st Street, San Diego, California 92105

First edition 1992

© 1992 Paula McGee

Typeset in 10 on 12 Sabon by Intype, London

Printed in Great Britain by St Edmundsbury Press Ltd, Bury St Edmunds, Suffolk

ISBN 0 412 44080 6   1 56593 065 7 (USA)

For Dave and Ellie

Contents

Acknowledgements

This book could not have been written without the assistance of many friends and colleagues who gave up their time to help me. I would particularly like to thank Bahadur Singh, Sharada Sugitherajah, Khun Pranee, Renee Adomat, and Judith Usiskin. If any inaccuracies have crept in, it is my fault and not theirs.

I have also been helped and advised over the years by my students, who have all made contributions to my teaching. A special thanks must also go to Graham Goulding at East London Polytechnic, who, with long-suffering patience, supervised the research from which this book was developed. This manuscript would never have left my desk without the help of Mandy Bridgewater who typed it.

Finally, I have to thank the many patients and their families who have encouraged me to learn, and to try to understand.

Preface

Perhaps I should begin by saying that I am not, in terms of ethnic origin, English. My parents emigrated to England from the Irish Republic, and we have all lived in Britain for so long that no one can see the join − or can they?

Some years ago, my mother was admitted to hospital for a routine operation. A ward nurse saw her obviously foreign name on the admissions list, and concluded she must be Asian. Accordingly, she arranged for my mother to have a bed in the same bay as other Asian women, and ordered her a curry for lunch.

Part of me was angry at the stereotypical thinking that everyone with a strange name must be Asian, but I had to concede that I myself knew little about other cultures. My own patients came from a variety of cultural traditions, but neither I nor my colleagues knew very much about them. What information we had was culled directly from patients and their families in a haphazard 'do this' or 'don't do that' basis. Because we had no understanding of the traditions, staff could become exasperated over what they interpreted as 'awkwardness'. Our inadequacies were further highlighted when patients did not speak English: there was always the question of who could translate for them, and whether they fully understood their illnesses and their treatments. For some, the experience of being in hospital must have been frightening.

On becoming a nurse tutor in 1980, I was surprised to find that no time was set aside to prepare students to care for patients from different cultural traditions, and I set out to remedy this situation. There was little published material on which to draw, no one to advise me, and I had no access to a proper academic library.

Between 1983–8 I introduced ideas on transcultural aspects of care into an RGN curriculum. I began with two three-hour sessions and gradually expanded the content into a programme of approximately 25 hours. Eventually, I was able to evaluate my efforts through completing my Master's dissertation.

This book is a reworking of that dissertation and represents a few small steps forward. It includes additional material for teachers, which I can honestly say from my experience has been successful in the classroom. It provides teachers with ideas that will enable them to include transcultural aspects of care in the curriculum by:

- presenting an overview of the issues involved in learning to care for people from different cultural backgrounds;
- discussing a variety of approaches for including transcultural care in the curriculum;
- proposing and discussing possible strategies that may assist the teacher in the classroom and the nurse in practice;
- offering further sources of information.

While the amount of published material about the care of people from various cultural traditions has increased markedly in recent years, there are still many aspects that receive little or no attention. There is, for example, a noticeable lack of contributions by members of ethnic minority groups; theirs are very small voices compared with those who write about cultures other than their own.

Although within nurse education there is now a considerable amount of research and other texts on the importance of the cultural dimensions of nursing and the content of curricula, there are far fewer examples of what might constitute good practice, or at least contribute to a debate about its nature. This book is intended as a beginning in addressing these issues.

ETHNIC MINORITIES

Culture is essentially a design for living (Allen, 1982); a way of life adopted by a particular group of people. It has two elements: the manifest dimension, that is, the aspects about people that can be observed, such as the things they make, how they cook, how they behave; and the tacit element, which includes values, attitudes, and beliefs. These are rarely explicit, and only traceable through the manifest aspects of a culture.

Cultures may be described as dominant or minority. A **dominant culture** is one that has, or assumes it has, the authority to act as guardian and sustainer of the controlling value system, and has a monopoly on the rewards available. A **minority culture** is one that possesses certain traits that are held in low esteem by the dominant culture. Those traits can be gender, as in the case of women; gender orientation, as in the case of homosexuality; race; ethnicity; profession; or some other characteristic that unites a group of people. The term minority has nothing to do with numbers. Women, for example, make up approximately half the total population of the world but may be described as a minority in relation to the dominant patriarchal culture (Khan, 1982; Tajfel, 1982).

'Ethnicity' describes a group of people who are clearly identifiable because of their way of life. Associated with this way of life may be factors such as religion, nationality or country of origin; and specific values, attitudes, or behaviour (Sorofman, 1986).

In this book, the term 'ethnic minority' is used to indicate people who do not belong to or identify with the dominant culture. It includes those who are Black as well as those who are not Black, depending on the cultural context.

REFERENCES

Allen, S. (1982) Perhaps a seventh person? *Women's Studies International Quarterly*, 3, 325–8. Reprinted in (ed. C. Husband) (1982) *Race in Britain*, Open Univ. Press.

Husband, C. see Khan, V. S. (1982).

Khan, V. S. (1982) Role of the culture of dominance in structuring the experience of ethnic minorities in *Race in Britain*, (ed. C. Husband), Open Univ. Press.

Sorofman, B. (1986) Research in cultural diversity. *Western J. of Nursing Research*, 8 (1), 121–3.

Tajfel, H. (1978) The social psychology of ethnic minorities, Minority Rights Group Report No. 38. Reprinted in *Race in Britain*, (ed. C. Husband) (1986) Open Univ. Press.

ONE

Issues in transcultural nursing

Teaching Transcultural Care: A guide for teachers of nursing and health care. Paula McGee. Published in 1992 by Chapman & Hall, London. ISBN 0 412 44080 6. © 1992 Paula McGee

Ms Chung has been admitted to hospital with a pelvic injury following a car accident. After being transferred from a trolley to a bed in the ward, the ward nurse begins to talk to her:

Nurse:	'Are you comfortable?'
Ms Chung:	Remains silent.
Nurse:	'Have you got a lot of pain?'
Ms Chung:	Looks away and makes no reply.
Nurse:	'I'll bring you some painkillers.'

The nurse brings some tablets to the bedside.

Nurse:	'These are quite strong. They'll help you to get some sleep too. Can you lift your head just a bit to take them?'
Ms Chung:	'No.'
Nurse:	'You can't lift your head?'
Ms Chung:	'No. No pills!'
Nurse:	'But they'll help get rid of the pain. Help you to sleep. You'll feel better if you take these. Come on.'
Ms Chung:	'No pills! No!' Looks distressed.
Nurse:	'Look, come on! It won't take a minute – they'll help you!'

Ms Chung continues to refuse to take the tablets and eventually the nurse goes away, taking the painkillers with her. She feels angry. In her opinion, Ms Chung is clearly in pain, so why won't she accept analgesia?

Ms Chung too is unhappy. For her, physical pain is a sign that something is wrong with her body – its natural balance and harmony have been disturbed, and must be restored. From what the nurse has said, Ms Chung thinks the painkillers will make her drowsy, clouding her consciousness and thus causing further disharmony in her body. She is upset and frightened by the nurse's behaviour.

Clearly, neither Ms Chung nor the nurse have communicated effectively, nor understood the other's point of view.

THE CODE OF PROFESSIONAL CONDUCT

Ms Chung's situation is not uncommon. Each patient/client brings to the health-care situation their own values, beliefs, and customs. The nurse, as a human being, brings to the same situation not only his or her own values, beliefs, and customs, but also those of the nursing profession. Inevitably, the stage is set for some potential misunderstanding between two, if not three, cultural systems.

It is the nurse who is charged with responsibility in this situation. The Code of Professional Conduct requires that he or she 'take account of the customs, values and spiritual beliefs of patients/clients' (UKCC, 1984).

While the phrase 'to take account of' is extremely broad, and there is a lack of clarity with regard to intent, evidence suggests that nurses take less account of their patients than might reasonably be expected. The central question remains, however, one of how individuals' values, beliefs, and customs are to be reflected in the delivery of nursing care.

In order to reach out to each patient and establish a therapeutic relationship, the nurse must have some knowledge and understanding of individual and cultural differences. We can begin to look at this by examining two key issues: racism, and transcultural nursing theory.

RACISM

It must be acknowledged that discussion about racism doubtless will raise a few eyebrows. Some may hold the view that it is inappropriate for nurses or other health-care workers to address racism. Leininger (1978), for example, devoted very little attention to the subject except to note that cultural diversity may be associated with colour, and that nurses with racist views may try to avoid transcultural nursing.

There is considerable evidence to support the view that members of the ethnic minorities receive inferior health-care services (Wright, 1983), and that one of the reasons for this is undoubtedly racism (NAHA, 1988; Evers et al., 1988). The National

Association of Health Authorities' (NAHA) report especially commented on the under-representation of ethnic minority people at all levels of decision-making in the NHS. The report recommended that this situation be addressed by: actively involving members of ethnic minority groups in all aspects of the health-care system; improving accessibility to the services by providing information in languages other than English; and by compiling a national database on the health education needs of Black and minority groups.

Health-care workers who are themselves members of ethnic minority groups may experience an additional form of discrimination. Hoffenburg (1985) commented on the high numbers of Black doctors who occupy junior posts in the less popular specialities such as geriatrics and psychiatry. The same trend, he observes, is to be found in nursing, a view confirmed by Baxter (1988), who found that Black nurses are denied opportunities in almost every situation.

The Commission for Racial Equality (1984) found that discrimination occurred in other fields as well, for example, an employment policy that discriminated against Black people at St Chad's Hospital in Birmingham, between 1973–9 was attributed to a domestic services manager. In the field of education and training, the lack of opportunities for ethnic minority staff means they will be under-represented on selection panels and in senior posts, thus confirming the message 'You can't achieve here.' Recruitment and selection processes, as well as curricula and syllabis are in urgent need of revision in order to provide a more multiracial and multicultural perspective (NAHA, 1988).

In this context, racism must be seen as an issue requiring urgent and sustained action if the quality of health-care services to ethnic minorities is to be improved; it is not good enough simply to omit it from education programmes because it means that some uncomfortable truths about the delivery of health care must be faced. Whilst Stenhouse (1982) asserted that any form of teaching about race relations will probably have a positive effect compared with no teaching at all, the manner in which racism is addressed is also very important if entrenched attitudes and stereotypes are to be effectively challenged. Is it possible for a teacher to honestly present to students the experiences of an ethnic minority group of which he or she is not a member? Can the teacher present the lived experience of being on the receiving-end of prejudice and discrimination? How can the teacher support ethnic minority students when, in sharing their experiences of discrimination, the dominant culture responds with, 'It's not true! You're exaggerating! You're making it all up.'?

There are no easy answers to these questions. The study of racism is not simply academic; it inevitably involves challenging attitudes and beliefs. Above all else, however, it must seek to be constructive, rather than an acrimonious dispute based on 'You do this!' versus 'No we don't!'

Racism can take many forms – discrimination against Gypsies, Jews, Irish (Curtis, 1971), Palestinians, Afro-Carribbean, to name only a few – and the teacher may need to consider which aspect of the subject he or she can most credibly address, either alone or with colleagues. Chapter 3 contains a quiz developed by the author in collaboration with a teacher colleague who is Black. We have used it together in class as a way of raising students' racial awareness. The quiz can be used as it stands, or as a basis for developing material to address other forms of discrimination.

THEORIES OF TRANSCULTURAL NURSING

The idea that culture is influential in nursing care is not new. Florence Nightingale (1894) was obviously aware of this when she wrote, 'It is a truism to say that the women who teach in India must know the language, the religions, superstitions and customs of the women to be taught in India. It ought to be a truism to say the very same for England.' The transcultural aspect of care, however, has been very neglected since Nightingale's time, and only recently have nurses begun to give it serious consideration. Predictably, different schools of thought have emerged.

Madeleine Leininger, an American nurse and anthropologist,

argues that the study of different cultures is essential for nurses if they are to gain an understanding of the similarities and differences between people. This is an essential prerequisite to developing insight into culturally determined patterns of socialization and styles of living; cultural dimensions of health and illness; and an awareness of self and others on which the provision of holistic care depends (Leininger, 1970, 1978).

Leininger sees this study as having two dimensions. First, there is a need for nurses to undertake studies in anthropology to develop a database of information about culturally determined aspects of health, illness, and care. Such databases would challenge the ethnocentric orientation of Western health-care systems, which insists their approaches are the only ones possible. Secondly, Leininger sees a need to address the application of this database to patient/client care. She developed a transcultural nursing theory, which she defines as,

> . . . a comparative analysis of different cultures and subcultures . . . with the goal of using this knowledge to provide culture-specific . . . nursing care to people [and which] reflects the synthesis of selected knowledge from anthropology and nursing and the development of new knowledge . . . to improve health care to people. . . . (Leininger, 1984)

Some unique features of Leininger's work include a focus on the concept of care as the distinguishing feature of nursing, setting it apart from other professions, notably medicine. Caring acts are universal, and may take many different forms, such as comforting, touching, physical care, etc., but the manner in which these acts are used, and the importance attached to them varies from one culture to another (Leininger 1981, 1985).

Leininger (1981) also takes into account the systems of treatment and care already extant within other cultures. She argues that these 'folk systems' need to be incorporated into professional approaches to care, which then might be aimed at assisting the individual in maintaining their existing health status and lifestyle; adapting to new circumstances; or making major lifestyle changes in a culturally acceptable manner.

There are a number of firsthand accounts by nurses that demonstrate the importance of Leininger's work. Rothenburger (1987), for example, in an account of her work in South America, describes how she came to understand the 'supernurse syndrome, that my values and beliefs are correct and take precedence over someone else's values'.

The importance of providing culturally acceptable health-care services cannot be overestimated. For nurses to impose their views on others is both offensive and unprofessional; there is then every possibility that patients/clients will seek to avoid contact with professionals, even at risk to themselves (Leininger 1978; Mares *et al.* 1985; Demissie, 1986; Parsons, 1987).

There are today a wide range of writers in the field of transcultural nursing in the United States, Britain, and Australia (Orque *et al.*, 1983; Bruni, 1988; Dobson, 1991), and a growing awareness among nurses. However, transcultural nursing is not without its critics. Alibhai (1986) draws attention to the risk of superficiality: there are so many cultures that no one can be expected to know them all, and the result may be an oversimplified clarifying and packaging of cultures. One lesson, about Islam for example, produces so-called 'experts', who expect every Moslem to think and act in the same way. Bruni (1988) also sees risks in stereotyping people because they belong to a cultural group. In her view it is not enough to focus on the culture itself; we must also consider the factors that influence it. Problems must be seen in the context in which they occur: a man's hostility towards his wife for going out to work, for example, may have little to do with the culture, but a great deal to do with financial constraints and the tension arising from these.

Tripp-Reimer and Dougherty (1985) criticize transcultural nursing and nursing anthropology for the 'inappropriate or inaccurate use of terms, concepts and methods originating in anthropology'. They are especially concerned about the imprecise use of the term 'culture', and the apparent lack of rigour in research studies. In their view, 'questions of accuracy must be addressed more thoroughly in qualitative studies'. Littlewood (1988) is critical of what she sees as Leininger's attempts to create a nursing speciality by setting up courses in transcultural care. Littlewood felt this establishes the nurse as an 'expert', distant from the patients/clients and serves to perpetuate the idea that people from ethnic minorities are different and always require specialist advice.

Alongside this criticism alternative approaches have emerged. Nancy Roper et al. (1985), see the patient/client as an individual who progresses through life on an independence/dependence continuum, and who performs a range of 'activities of living'. Each of these activities can be affected by physical, environmental, and politico-economic, psychological, and socio-cultural factors. Thus the activity of communicating involves physiological elements such as speech and hearing; psychological elements such as personality and motivation; socio-cultural dimensions such as language and customs; environmental factors such as noise; and politico-economic factors such as the availability of communication resources. It could therefore be argued that Roper et al.'s approach allows for the consideration of ethnic differences at each stage without making them a 'special case'.

Ethnic minority people do not want to be singled out as different, but to be accepted as they are. While this theory may be valid, the model has been widely used in nursing in Britain in recent years with no noticeable improvement in the delivery of health care to members of ethnic minority groups. This is not necessarily due to a weakness in the theory, since variations in practice seem to be limitless. Many wards and departments use the activities of living, but fewer incorporate the other aspects of the model into their care systems. The result is that in practice, cultural factors will either be ignored, or will encourage the view that 'we do it anyway', which usually means 'we don't'.

In contrast, Sands and Hale (1988), while acknowledging the influence of Leininger's work, adopt a different approach to meeting the health-care needs of ethnic minorities. In their view, within American society there is a culture of poverty that includes 'the aged, the alcoholic, the inner-city poor, the rural poor, farm workers, migrants and the ethnic groups'. They recognize that this concept of a 'culture of poverty' is contentious, but argue that the poor are frequently dehumanized by the health-care system. The process by which this dehumanization occurs includes 'viewing clients as things or problems, seeing clients as inferior and unworthy of attention and denying clients choices'. As Curtis (1971), amongst others, has demonstrated, this process of dehumanization occurs also in racism. Those who are the object of prejudice are frequently represented as having animal-like qualities or as beasts. Health-care workers therefore need help in examining their attitudes and prejudices towards people who are poor in order to identify and change those factors that contribute to dehumanized care.

While this may be easier said than done, Sand's and Hale's work suggests opportunities for nurses to develop both personally and professionally, rather than becoming 'experts', who may not be available when the patient's/client's needs are greatest.

SUMMARY

In developing an approach to the teaching of transcultural care, the author has brought together different theoretical perspectives in order to enable students to develop a sound knowledge-base about local ethnic minorities; to reappraise their attitudes; and to apply the understanding gained to patient care.

A number of issues have been examined, including racism; the question of whether the nurse should become an 'expert' who emerges as a result of academic study; the misuse of approaches to nursing that could help nurses in practice; and a focus on the 'culture of poverty' shared by a number of different groups in society. These issues have been used in developing the teaching package in Chapters 3 and 4.

REFERENCES

Alibhai, Y. (1986) Can't they see I'm me. *Nursing Times*, **82**, 56.
Baxter, C. (1988b) The black nurse: an endangered species. A case for equal opportunities in nursing, Training in Health and Race.

Bruni, N. (1988) A critical analysis of transcultural theory. *Australian J. of Advanced Nursing*, 15 (3), 26–36.

Comm. for Racial Equality (1984) *St Chad's Hospital – Report of a Formal Investigation.* Comm. for Racial Equality.

Demissie, A. (1986) Health and social services: the cultural obstacles. *Geriatric Medicine* 16 (11), 53–4.

Dobson, S. (1983) Bringing culture into care. *Nursing Times*, Feb. 9, 53–7.

Dobson, S. (1991) *Transcultural Nursing – A Contemporary Imperative*, Scutari.

Evers, H. *et al.* (1988) *Community Care Working Papers*, Dept. of Social Medicine, Birmingham Univ.

Hoffenburg, Sir R. (1985) National Health Service: race and health report on a lecture. *The Lancet*, Feb. 16, 410–11.

Leininger, M. (1970) *Nursing and Anthropology: Two Worlds to Blend*, John Wiley, New York.

Leininger, M. (1978) *Transcultural Nursing: Concepts, Theories and Practices*, John Wiley, New York.

Leininger, M. (1981) Transcultural nursing: its progress and its future. *Nursing and Health Care*, 2 (7), 365–71.

Leininger, M. (1984a) *Care: the Essence of Nursing and Health*, Wayne State Univ. Press, Detroit.

Leininger, M. (1985) Transcultural nursing diversity and universality: a theory of nursing. *Nursing and Health Care*, 6 (4), 209–12.

Littlewood, J. (1988) The patient's world. *Nursing Times*, 84 (3), 29–30.

Mares, P., Henley, A. and Baxter, C. (1985) *Health Care in Multiracial Britain*, Health Education Council and National Extension College.

National Assoc. of Health Authorities (1988) *Action not words: a strategy to improve health services for black and minority ethnic groups*, National Assoc. of Health Authorities.

Nightingale, F. (1894) Health teaching in towns and villages, rural hygiene, in Bringing culture into care, S. Dobson (1983), *Nursing Times*, Feb. 9, 53–7.

Orque, M., Bloch, B. and Monrroy, L. (1983) *Ethnic Nursing Care*, C. V. Mosby.

Parsons, L. (1987) Flexible care strategies, *Health Service J.*, Feb. 19, 214–15.

Roper, N., Logan, W. and Tierney, A. (1985) *The Elements of Nursing*, Churchill Livingstone.

Rothenburger, R. (1987) Understanding cultural differences is the key to transcultural nursing. *AORN J.*, **45** (5), 1203–8.

Sands, R. and Hale, S. (1988) Enhancing cultural sensitivity in clinical practice. *J. of the National Black Nurses Association*, **2** (1), 54–63.

Stenhouse, L. *et al.* (1982) *Teaching About Race Relations: Problems and Effects*, Routledge and Kegan Paul. Slightly adapted and abridged in *Multicultural Education: Principles and Practice*, Lynch, J. (1986), Routledge and Kegan Paul.

Tripp-Reimer, T. and Dougherty, M. (1985) Cross-cultural nursing research. *Annual Review of Nursing Research*, **3**, 77–104.

United Kingdom Central Council for Nursing, Midwifery and Health Visiting (1984) *Code of Professional Conduct*, UKCC.

Wright, C. M. (1983) Language and communication problems in the Asian community, *J. of the Royal College of General Practitioners*, Feb., 101–4.

TWO

Testing the water: multicultural education today

Teaching Transcultural Care: A guide for teachers of nursing and health care. Paula McGee. Published in 1992 by Chapman & Hall, London. ISBN 0 412 44080 6. © 1992 Paula McGee

This chapter examines the practical issues involved in curriculum development. Ideas from nursing literature and general education have been used to develop some broad guidelines, which are divided into two groups. The general points are mainly concerned with developing the curriculum to include transcultural nursing; the specific points deal with content and style.

MULTICULTURAL EDUCATION

Multicultural education in Britain appears to be in a constant state of flux, and there is a lack of clarity about what is and is not acceptable practice. Lynch (1986) identifies five distinct phases, none of which seems to have gained wholehearted support.

The *'laissez-faire'* phase lasted from approximately the end of the Second World War until the early 1960s. It was characterized by a belief in the supremacy of British culture and ignorance of others, including the new groups entering the country. The second phase, 'English as a second language', saw the development of the notion that immigrants newly arrived in Britain had only to learn to speak English in order to be fully assimilated into British society.

In the mid-1970s it became clear that this simplistic approach would not do. There was a growing awareness of the problems faced by members of ethnic minorities. During the third, 'deficit', phase emphasis was placed on valuing different lifestyles and on enhancing the self-esteem of ethnic-minority members. From the late 1970s this approach broadened into the 'multicultural' phase, in which wider issues such as curriculum design and content, teaching strategies and assessment, were addressed alongside ideas from the previous phase.

The true multicultural curriculum was seen as 'a process whereby the individual develops competencies in multiple cultural systems utilized to generate standards for perceiving, evaluating, believing and doing' (Lynch, 1983). Jeffcoate (1976) argues that the multicultural curriculum should promote an awareness of one's own culture, thus reinforcing a sense of identity and pride in oneself. However, Jeffcoate also states that the multicultural curriculum should not prevent acculturation, the process whereby one culture adapts features from another; 'The preservation of minority cultures in a fossilized form is not what multicultural education should be doing' (Jeffcoate, 1976). Such statements continued to fuel the debate about multicultural education. During recent years there has been, as Lynch puts it, 'mounting politicization of multicultural education from both the right and the left'. This is largely because to the one it appears too radical and to the other not radical enough. Out of this has arisen the fifth phase in multicultural education, which is concerned with anti-racism. This continues alongside the multicultural phase in an attempt to tackle prejudice and racism in schools.

CURRICULUM MODELS

In the field of transcultural care, Byerly (1977) outlines four curriculum models:

1 The integrative approach is one in which 'cultural concepts and constructs are unified . . . with other content . . . in such a manner that students are encouraged to discover, create and think about rather than accumulate, more facts'. In other words, transcultural concepts pervade the whole curriculum.

2 In the unit-construction approach, 'specific learning units . . . deal primarily with cultural components in health and nursing care'. Thus, each aspect of the curriculum, for example maternity care or care of the elderly, may have a specific unit of study on transcultural concepts related to that area.

3 The course approach requires 'educationally prepared faculty (with a background in anthropology) to provide a concentrated emphasis on cultural aspects in health and illness'.

4 Finally, the interdisciplinary approach 'introduces cultural components in conjunction with classes offered by departments of anthropology or social science'.

Byerly's ideas may be usefully compared with those of mainstream multicultural education. The integrative approach may at first seem ideal, and may be equated with Lynch's 'permeation' approach. However, Lynch argues that this will involve redesigning the entire curriculum, a difficult task if the teacher lacks experience in multicultural education; furthermore, staff may feel threatened by such an upheaval. Burrows (1983) also sees the influence of the teacher as crucial in this approach in that the 'information given . . . is likely to be subject to the influence of ethnocentrism . . . and care must be taken to avoid superficiality in using this approach'.

The unit-instruction approach closely resembles Lynch's 'additive tactics', in which small units are added to the existing curriculum to broaden knowledge. Lynch regards this as 'tokenism in that such units tend to be superficial thus leaving the pupils' knowledge-base unchanged'. Burrows sees unit instruction as a repetitive and time-consuming approach. In her view, there is a danger that ethnic differences may be over-emphasized and seen as problems.

The course approach may be seen to correspond with Lynch's 'parallel tactics', in which separate units of study are set up outside the main curriculum. An example of this might be 'Black studies'. Leininger (1978) sees the course approach as highly appropriate for qualified nurses; higher degrees in transcultural care are essential in the production of 'experts'. Lynch and Burrows both regard this approach as undesirable, simply because it places transcultural work outside the main curriculum, unrelated to other areas, and thus of low prestige.

Lynch also describes a 'materials production' approach, which usually involves a teaching package such as a race training-pack, which is essentially knowledge-based. This is not a feature of transcultural nursing so far. Lynch does not appear to favour any particular approach, but he does indicate this might prove to be a useful starting place for introducing multicultural work into the curriculum. He advises that the teacher should begin in a small way in order to overcome any difficulties and to gain acceptance of the subject area.

Byerly appears to favour a combination of approaches: 'A combination of three of them seems most desirable: integration of cultural components at all levels . . . at least one distinct course on cultural diversity in health and illness plus supporting interdisciplinary social science or anthropology courses'. She goes on to point out that what is possible depends ultimately on the 'size and educational preparation of faculty, available resources . . . the level at which students enter the nursing programme [and] the degree of voluntary or required affirmative action to meet the needs of various ethnic/minority groups'.

CURRICULUM CONTENT

There would appear to be no ideal approach to the teaching of transcultural care. The first consideration must be what is practicable, particularly in relation to pre-registration or part-time students, whose classroom time is limited. Some of the strategies outlined in the literature are intended for full-time, post-registration courses in transcultural care. Gunter (1988), for example, took her students to Jamaica for the experience of living and working in another culture – a venture clearly beyond the resources of most teachers.

The amount of time available needs to be considered realistically. The teaching package outlined in Chapter 3 requires approximately five classroom sessions spread over a number of weeks. The second part of the package, in Chapter 4, requires more time, depending on which exercises are selected by the teacher, and needs to be spread out over several weeks.

The concept of culture should be addressed, together with an examination of the stereotypes and genuine differences that may exist between groups (Mattson, 1987). The nurse should develop an increased awareness of his or her own culture (Tuck and Harris, 1988) as well as that of the profession (Leininger, 1978) in order to become sensitive to the interface between these and others.

It is neither practical nor desirable to attempt to teach students about many different cultures; the aims should rather be on developing a set of principles that equip the nurse to care for people not just of one culture but of many different ones. Developing an awareness of his or her own culture will enable the nurse to examine issues such as prejudice, discrimination, values, beliefs, attitudes, and social mores. Ideas about health and illness and the expectations people may have of professionals can also be explored and compared. The culture of Western professional health care also should be examined and compared with that of other cultures (Leininger 1978, 1981) so that nurses are made aware of the potential for culture clash and culture shock (Baxter, 1988a).

The principles of communication across cultural boundaries is a neglected area in transcultural nursing literature. And yet, if the nurse and the patient cannot communicate effectively, misunderstandings arise and patients receive inferior health care (Wright, 1983; Watson, 1985; NAHA 1988). Finally, the nurse must be able to apply the knowledge and understanding gained in the care of patients: assessment is the major skill area (Chapter 4).

Multicultural education offers a different, less prescriptive approach to content. Jeffcoate sees multicultural education as being largely concerned with education of attitudes, beliefs, and feelings. A certain amount of specific knowledge and skill is in his view desirable, but of lesser importance than the concept of respect for others and for oneself.

The achievement of respect for others lies in knowledge. For example, as Jeffcoate says, all pupils should, 'know and understand the basic facts of race difference . . . and should be able to recognize racism and other forms of prejudice and should accept the unique value of every human being and the principles of equal rights and justice for all.'

The concept of respect for self is achieved in a similar way, and while Jeffcoate expresses his ideas using the format of behavioural objectives, he also acknowledges their limitations. In the affective domain there is no 'right answer', and in this view multicultural education is essentially concerned with attitudes, beliefs, and feelings.

TEACHING STRATEGIES

Jeffcoate and Lynch expand on these ideas in the discussion of teaching strategies in multicultural education. Again, there appears to be no 'right' approach. Jeffcoate makes the distinction between a 'transmissionist' style, in which the pupil accepts whatever the teacher says, and a 'transformationist' style in which the pupil is encouraged to question and to criticize.

Lynch feels the key to teaching strategies is the notion of respect for pupils. To achieve this the teacher must be aware of his or her own biases, and have a knowledge of cultural groups. This should enable the teacher to become aware of culturally defined behaviour, such as showing acceptance and feeling; and to encourage co-operation and different communication styles. The teacher must be willing to 'unlearn' something every day.

In transcultural nursing theory, the teaching strategies, where they are described, are open and student-centred. For example, Gould-Stuart (1986) describes a programme conducted in a home for the elderly where the residents were mainly Jewish and the staff came from another cultural group. The aim was to modify a 'them-and-us' situation that had arisen between the staff and the residents. A series of seminars lasting ten weeks explored various aspects of ageing with reference to other cultures. The examples used were drawn from cultures outside the everyday experience of the staff, thus preventing a sense of being threatened or criticized. The stereotype of the uncaring family was explored, and role-play was used to illustrate cross-cultural misunderstandings.

Stern (1985) describes her programme in Louisiana, where she herself was perceived by students as being from another culture – the San Francisco Bay area. She introduced ideas about cultural differences very gradually in three distinct stages. First she describes 'testing the water', in which culture was discussed without any specific references. In the second phase, 'making a splash', transcultural nursing theory was introduced. Finally, 'heading for shore' involved the analysis of the data she had collected while introducing transcultural nursing into the curriculum. Her teaching strategies included role-play and gaming, as well as inviting people who were happy to discuss their culture with the students. In encouraging the students to take an active part in the development of course materials, Stern believes a situation of shared learning between herself and the students resulted in greater mutual respect.

SUMMARY

In introducing transcultural care into the curriculum, a number of educational approaches are possible. It would seem to be best to begin in a small way, and to reinforce the teaching at intervals throughout the course. Curriculum content should cover a range of issues in the cognitive and affective domains, and the nurse should be able to apply the understanding gained to direct patient/client care. Teaching strategies need to be open and student-centred in order to create opportunities for both personal and professional development.

The remainder of the book is essentially a teaching package, which demonstrates how transcultural care can be introduced into the curriculum. Ideas for teaching at different stages are included, as well as strategies for evaluation and assessment.

REFERENCES

Baxter, C. (1988a) Culture shock. *Nursing Times*, **84** (2), 36–8.

Burrows, A. (1983) Patient-centred nursing care in a multi-racial society: the relevance of ethnographic perspectives in nursing curricula. *J. of Advanced Nursing*, **8**, 477–85.

Byerly, E. (1977) Cultural components in the baccalaureate nursing curriculum – philosophy goals and processes in *National League for Nursing*, Cultural dimensions in the baccalaureate nursing curriculum: workshop papers. National League for Nursing.

Gould-Stuart, J. (1986) Bridging the cultural gap between residents and staff. *Geriatric Nursing*, Nov/Dec, 319–21.

Gunter, L. M. (1988) Notes on a method for teaching transcultural nursing, in *Recent Advances in Nursing: Issues in Cross-Cultural Nursing*, (ed. J. M. Morse), Churchill Livingstone.

Jeffcoate, R. (1976) Curriculum planning in multicultural education. *Educational Research*, **18** (3), 192–200.

Leininger, M. (1978) *Transcultural Nursing: Concepts, Theories and Practices*, John Wiley, New York.

Leininger, M. (1981) Transcultural nursing: its progress and its future. *Nursing and Health Care*, **2** (7), 365–71.

Lynch, J. (1983) *The Multicultural Curriculum*, Batsford Academic and Educational Ltd, London.

Lynch, J. (1986) *Multicultural Education: Principles and Practice*, Routledge and Kegan Paul.

Mattson, S. (1987) The need for cultural concepts in the nursing curriculum. *J. of Nursing Education*, **26** (5), 206–8.

Morse, J. (ed.) (1988) *Recent Advances in Nursing: Issues in Cross-Cultural Nursing*, Churchill Livingstone.

National Assoc. of Health Authorities (1988) *Action not words: a strategy to improve health services for black and minority ethnic groups*, National Assoc. of Health Authorities.

National League for Nursing (1977) *Curriculum dimensions in the baccalaureate nursing curriculum: workshop papers*, National League for Nursing.

Poulter, S. (1986) *English law and ethnic minority customs*, Butterworth, London.

Stern, P. (1985) Teaching transcultural nursing in Louisiana from the ground up. *Health Care for Women International*, **6** (1–3), 175–86.

Tuck, I. and Harris, L. H. (1988) Teaching students transcultural concepts. *Nurse Educator*, **13** (3), 36–9.

Watson, P. (1985) Tower of Bable. *Nursing Times*, Dec. 3, 40–1.

Wright, C. M. (1983) Language and communication problems in the Asian community, *J. of the Royal College of General Practitioners*, Feb., 101–4.

THREE

Transcultural care through self-awareness

Teaching Transcultural Care: A guide for teachers of nursing and health care. Paula McGee. Published in 1992 by Chapman & Hall, London. ISBN 0 412 44080 6. © 1992 Paula McGee

This chapter is essentially a teaching package that is aimed at introducing the subject of transcultural care. It is suitable for both qualified nurses who have received no previous teaching on this subject, and pre-registration students during their foundation course.

Four topic areas are presented: cultural self-awareness; equal opportunities; communication; and health and illness. Each topic is explored through the use of different activities, for example, questionnaires or role-plays. While the topics and activities do not need to be used in any particular order, and may be selected at random, it is advisable to cover all of the topics as they are interrelated.

The activities are intended both to form and to stimulate discussion about each individual's own culture and preferences and to stimulate an awareness of both inter- and intracultural differences. While most of the activities can be completed by working alone, the reader will find that they lend themselves more readily to groupwork.

There is enough material for five sessions at least; ideally it should be spread over a number of weeks to allow students time to reflect on what has been discussed.

QUESTIONNAIRE: CULTURAL SELF-AWARENESS

Give each member of the group a copy of the questionnaire below, and ask them to answer each question in the spaces provided. Time: 10–15 minutes.

1 *List six words/phrases that you think describe you.*

What, in your opinion, are your strengths?

What, in your opinion, are your main achievements so far?

2   *With which societies do you associate the following games?*
    mah-jong   hurley
    derrah   cricket
    baseball   mutorere

3 *Write down your full name, including title (Mr, Mrs, Ms, etc.)*

What information does this name convey to others about you?

How does your name change with the following:
   formal occasions
   polite but informal occasions
   for use only by a close friend or relative
   impolite or rude situations

4 *When you are introduced to someone for the first time do*
   you:
     shake hands
     smile and look at the other person or at the floor
     embrace
     kiss
     bow

What factors influence your behaviour in this situation?

In what ways would your behaviour differ if you were to meet a friend or relative?

5   *What do you most like to eat and drink?*

What do you least like to eat and drink?

Is there something you would never consider eating or drinking under any circumstances? Why?

6   *At the end of the day, do you like to relax in a long, hot bath, or to take a shower?*

•

ANSWERS

There are no right answers to this questionnaire, but the following points may help to promote discussion.

Question 1

This question asks you to focus on how you see yourself, and to identify your strengths and achievements. You may have written statements such as, 'I am good at . . .', 'I see myself as . . .'. Some people are by nature reticent, and find it difficult to make statements which begin with 'I'. In Britain, statements such as 'I am good at . . .' may be considered a form of bragging, and yet Western societies generally encourage a focus on the individual. This is not universally shared. Harrington (1988) describes Guatemalan women whose sense of identity is group rather than individually orientated. Benner and Wrubel (1989) argue that the cult of individuality fosters 'negative freedom', which restricts the person's ability to choose and to relate to others.

Question 2

Ideas about what is enjoyable vary not only from one individual to another, but also from one society to another. These games are not played exclusively by the people of the countries listed below, but are associated with them:

mah-jong, China   cricket, Britain, West Indies,
derrah, Nigeria   India, Pakistan
baseball, United States   mutorere, New Zealand (Maori)
hurley, Ireland

Question 3

Our Western naming systems convey information about our gender, family, and, in the case of women, marital status. The individual's age may also be indicated by his or her first names, as these tend to be subject to fashion.

Other naming systems differ greatly. For example, a name may indicate a person's religion but not their marital status or even their gender. The Western convention of the first name followed by the surname, usually given in this order, may not apply. Below are some examples of other naming systems.

Sikh names have three components. First names, such as Darjinder, Harvinder, and Dlbeiro, are used by family and friends. The same names are used for men and women. Middle names indicate that the person is a Sikh. All women have the name Kaur meaning 'princess', and all men have the name Singh, meaning 'lion-hearted'. Sometimes people omit their religious name, but others may use it as a surname. The family name, such as Gill or Dhillon, may sometimes be omitted. Sikh names may therefore have several variations. Ravinder Singh Gill, for example, may be the same person as Ravinder Gill, or Ravinder Singh. His wife may be Baljit Kaur Gill, Baljit Gill, or Baljit Kaur. Health-care workers will need to ascertain an individual's full name, and, in the absence of a family name, those of close relatives. When addressing a Sikh person it is polite to use his or her full name.

Moslem names have different systems for men and women because in Islamic tradition they are separate. Men's names include a religious name, such as Mohammed, which indicates that the person is a Moslem; a personal name such as Safdar, for use by family and friends; and a family name such as Hussain. The religious and personal names may be used in any order, and the family name may be omitted. Thus, Mohammed Aktar may be the same person as Aktar Mohammed. Women's names include a personal name, such as Amina or Nasreen; and a second name, which may be a title, such as Begum or Bibi. Alternatively, a woman may have two personal names. A woman may use her names in any order, and is not obliged to adopt the family name of either her father or her husband. In the absence of shared family names, health-care workers will need to ascertain both the name of the patient/client and those of close relatives. When addressing a Moslem person it is polite to use his or her full name.

In **Thailand**, names are chosen with great care. A baby's horoscope, and the date and time of birth, must all be considered. Advice will be sought from a monk, who will give the parents several appropriate names from which to choose. Each individual therefore has a first name, which has a special meaning, such as Nittaya, Puang Phen (in Thai, Ph is pronounced 'P', not 'F' as in English), and Duang Chan which are all girls' names associated with the moon, and a family name which also has a special meaning. The order in which the names are used is the same as in the Western tradition, but the family name is often not used. Instead, the first name is used for all official purposes, and each person has a nickname, which is used within the family. It is polite to use the first name preceded by Khun, thus Khun Nittaya, both when speaking and writing to a Thai person. At the age of fifteen a Thai is considered to be an adult, and it is appropriate to use adult terms of address in English – Mr, Mrs, Ms.

Question 4

In Britain, it is generally accepted that formal introductions will probably be accompanied by handshaking, smiling, and mutual gazing. However, physical contact may not be part of the social norms in other societies; smiling and mutual gazing may also be considered inappropriate. Below are some examples of other ways of greeting.

To greet as Hindus do, stand up straight, place your feet with the heels together, press the palms of your hands together in front of you at about the height of your breastbone, and say 'Nameste' (Nah-mest-ay). This formal greeting can be used when meeting or when leaving. Physical contact, especially between members of the opposite sex, is not considered appropriate. In informal situations it is acceptable to simply smile and say hello. People of the same gender who know each other well may embrace.

The formal greeting for Thais is very similar to that of the Hindu tradition, but the greeting is 'Sawadee'. Only women bow when making this greeting, in order to emphasize their femininity. A younger person should greet an elder first out of politeness. Among people who are Westernized, it is appropriate to shake hands.

Question 5

It is easy to stereotype ethnic groups in terms of the food they eat: the British eat fish and chips; Indians eat curry, and so on. The subject of food is probably one area in which health-care workers require the most knowledge – and cause the most offence. It is not enough, for example, to take the ham off the salad and expect the Jewish patient to eat it; nor is it enough to try to avoid the issue by writing 'Asian diet', 'kosher', or 'vegetarian' on the patient's menu card and then leave it up to the kitchen staff.

Religious beliefs strongly influence many people's choice of food, and the health-care worker needs a sound knowledge of what food an individual can eat and why, as well as how it should be prepared and served. The most obvious source of this information is the patient/client and their family. Set out below are some examples as illustrations.

Hindus believe it is wrong to take life, and most are therefore vegetarians. Strict Hindus will not eat any meat, fish, eggs, or cheese made with animal rennet. The degree to which these beliefs are observed will vary from one individual to another, and between castes.

In many Hindu homes, food is prepared so as to be eaten with the fingers. Only the right hand is used for serving food or passing a plate of food along the table; it also is the only hand used for eating and placing food in the mouth. Drinks may be held in the left hand, but not food. To offer food, or anything else, with the left hand is considered rude, because the left hand is used for toilet purposes.

For Jews, food must be kosher, that is, 'fit to eat'. Jewish dietary laws specify in detail those foods which are acceptable for human consumption – for example fish with scales and fins; poultry; meat from mammals with cloven hoofs – and those which are not, for example pork or shellfish. In addition to being kosher, food must be prepared and cooked in accordance with the laws and customs of *kashrut*. Meat and milk foods must be kept separate, and separate cooking utensils, crockery, and cutlery are used. These will be washed and dried separately, using a different washing-up bowl and tea-towel. Meat and milk are never served at the same meal, or within three hours of each other. Thus it would be inappropriate to offer coffee or tea with milk after a meal containing meat.

The majority of Thai people are Buddhist, and many prefer to be vegetarian. Meat and animal products are permissible provided the animal(s) were not killed solely for food. Buddhist monks and nuns in certain religious orders will eat only once a day, before noon. After that they may take only fluids, but without milk. In other orders monks and nuns may eat twice a day. Lay Thais are more relaxed about when they eat.

Table manners are informal within the Thai family. Food is normally eaten with a spoon and fork. An individual bowl is provided for each person to wash their hands during the meal. It is polite to leave a little food on the plate: when the person has finished eating, the remaining food is gathered to one side of the plate, and the spoon and fork are placed together. Outside the family, manners may be slightly more formal in that guests may wait to be served rather than help themselves, and they will not leave the table before their hosts. Men will sit cross-legged, but women will sit with their legs to one side, with the soles of their feet tucked out of sight so they are not pointing towards anyone, which is considered ill-mannered, as are sounds like burping or making noises while eating.

Question 6

The way in which people maintain their personal hygiene is a very private matter. Some will prefer a shower to a bath, or vice-versa. However, there may be more to consider than a simple matter of choice, as the following examples demonstrate:

Baths are not a feature of Indian homes in the subcontinent, and most people prefer a shower. While some will be happy to use a Western-style shower, others will prefer to stand or squat in the empty bath, and with a cup or jug pour water over themselves. Help will be accepted from a member of the same sex, although most people will not undress fully in front of anyone, even a member of the same sex. Some may even wear an undergarment while showering, drying and dressing in stages to preserve their modesty. Threads are often worn around the wrists or neck or other parts of the body; these are of sacred significance, and should never be removed.

In Thai homes, showers are preferred to baths. While some may use a Western-style shower, others will prefer to stand or to squat in the empty bath and pour water over themselves. If a bath is felt to be necessary, the Thai will want to wash before getting in to the bath, and will take a shower afterwards.

A Thai will always wash from the head down, and use at least two flannels – one for the head and the other for the body. A third may be kept for washing the feet, which are considered 'dirty'. It is very impolite to touch a person's head or face immediately after touching their feet, especially if the person is elderly. Most people will never undress fully either in front of anyone or alone. Carers must be of the same sex as there is a strong sense of individual privacy and dignity, even in close personal relationships.

Table 3.1 Equal opportunities quiz

Each member of the group is given a copy of the quiz and asked to work through it alone, indicating their answers by ticking the appropriate column. Time: 5 minutes.

		Fact	Fiction
1.	There is controlled immigration into Britain.	_____	_____
2.	Britain is becoming overcrowded as a result of immigration	_____	_____
3.	Issuing British passports to Hong Kong Chinese will cause a dramatic rise in the population in Britain.	_____	_____
4.	Immigration into Britain will increase in 1992.	_____	_____
5.	At least 40% of Black people were born in Britain.	_____	_____
6.	Black people are always cared for by their families, so they do not need the community nursing services.	_____	_____
7.	In the NHS, Black staff have fewer chances of promotion than White staff.	_____	_____
8.	There has been active recruitment of staff from abroad to fill vacancies in the NHS.	_____	_____
9.	The NHS does not take into account the health needs of ethnic minority people.	_____	_____
10.	An equal opportunities policy will end discrimination.	_____	_____

ANSWERS

Question 1

Fact. Since 1978 immigration to Britain has been greatly restricted (Fransman, 1982), see question 3.

Question 2

Fiction. During the early 1980s, the number of people emigrating from Britain annually exceeded those coming to live here, but during the period 1985–9 this trend was reversed, when more migrants entered Britain than left (Social Trends, 1991). Despite this trend, there is no evidence that Britain is becoming overcrowded as a result.

Question 3

Fiction. Not everyone who obtains a British passport may want to come to Britain; not all British passports entitle the bearer to live in Britain. There are different types of British passport, one for each classification of British citizenship: British citizenship; British dependent territories citizenship; British overseas citizenship; and citizen of commonwealth country. Individuals in the last three categories do not have the automatic right to live in Britain (Fransman, 1982).

Question 4

Fiction. In 1992, barriers between the member states of the European Community were removed. There is, however, no evidence to suppose this will cause the population of Britain to rise (see above).

Question 5

Fact. There have been Black people living in Britain for centuries, as evidenced in literature, such as *Vanity Fair* and *Othello*.

Question 6

Fiction. According to Evers, *et al.* (1988) Black families face many pressures in common with White families, yet receive less help from many community services, including community nurses.

Question 7

Fact. Baxter (1988a) found considerable evidence of racism against Black nurses at all levels of the profession.

Question 8

Fact. Recruitment began in 1948 when the NHS was established. Offices were opened in a number of British colonies, such as Nigeria, Mauritius, and Trinidad, through which staff were recruited as a solution to manpower shortages in Britain. This pattern of overseas recruitment continued for many years, but as Kushnick (1988) states, many people found that on arrival in Britain their jobs were very low in status, and opportunities to improve their lot were often barred by discrimination.

Question 9

Fact. The NAHA report, *Action Not Words* (1988) states clearly that the health needs of ethnic minorities are not being met, and that ethnic minority people are unrepresented in senior posts in the health service. Evers (1988) also found that ethnic minority people are least likely to receive help from the community nursing and other services, either because they are not informed about them or not referred to them. The myth that Black families always cope without outside help is still widely believed; there is also evidence of racism.

Question 10

Fiction. A policy is essentially a statement of intent on behalf of an organization. It is the use of the policy by the people in an organization that will determine its success.

COMMUNICATION

Students should be asked to work in small groups to attempt these role-play situations. Each group can then explore the issues which arise, rather than just passively watch. Students will need to be briefed at least one week in advance if they are to participate effectively. Students who have some knowledge, however elementary, of another language may find it useful in undertaking these exercises but this knowledge is not essential. If video equipment is available, a recording of the students' attempts at the role-play situations will form a useful basis for the ensuing discussion and debriefing.

Role-play 1 – getting help

Briefing for patient

You are abroad, visiting a country where you do not speak the language very fluently. You are not feeling well, and decide to visit the local hospital. It is very large, and you feel very lost. Eventually you arrive in what seems to be a clinic. A member of staff approaches you with a form. You sit down with the person and try to answer the questions.

Briefing for nurse

It is a very busy morning in the clinic and you are rushed off your feet. Yet another new patient arrives to be clerked in. You begin asking the questions, but are called away. You give the form to the patient, asking him or her to fill it in. (Role-playing instruction: give the 'patient' the form in German and retain the English translation for your own use.)

When you come back, he or she has not answered the questions correctly, and has missed some out altogether. You tear up the form and start again. You then discover the patient does not speak your language fluently. What are you going to do?

Table 3.2   Rolle – spielen bekommen hilfe!

Kranke Kurzbiographie

Namen:

Addresse:

Telefon Nummer:

Datum von Geburstag: Aller:

Einlab Datum:

Grund von Einlab:

Tatigkeit:

Arzt Namen:
   Addresse:

Allergisch gegen:

Nachste Verwandschlaf:

Verwandte:

Namen:

Addresse:

Telefon Nummer:

Wollen sie ihren verwandte Benachrictigung?

Welcher tabletten sich haben?

Welcher Wertroll sich haben?
(beschreibend)

Table 3.3 Role play 1 – getting help

Patient Profile

Name:

Address:

Telephone No.:

Date of Birth: Age:

Admission Date:

Reason for Admission:

Occupation:

GP Name and Address:

Allergies:

Past Medical History:

Next of Kin: Relationship:

Address: Telephone No.:

Do you wish them to be notified?

What tablets have you been taking?

Have you brought any valuables? (Describe)

Debriefing

The purpose of this exercise is to demonstrate how misunder-standings can arise when people do not share a common language fully. The use of German is deliberate, because there are some similarities between German and English; however, perhaps because of this, the patient or nurse may think he/she has understood the question when in fact they have not.

In discussing this role-play, a number of points may arise. Those that relate to working in situations in which the patient and the health-care worker do not share the same language are summarized below.

- In this situation, because it would probably take longer than normal to conduct an interview, it would be appropriate to set aside more time at the beginning (Mareo, 1985).
- Tearing up the form is guaranteed to have a devastating effect on the patient's morale and self-esteem.
- The nurse's voice may have become raised during the interview, betraying irritation and perhaps the feeling that the client/patient is shamming. In a real situation, this of course would be counter-productive.
- The complexity of ideas presented to the patient may add to their difficulty in responding. In analysing the role-play, examine how the ideas are grouped together, and how these might be separated to make answering easier.
- Jargon and colloquialisms can further complicate the matter. It is best to avoid them and to use simple (Bal, 1981) words and phrases that are easily understood.
- Pay attention to non-verbal communication as well; the patient/client may be trying to say something without using words.
- The nurse may also give information non-verbally. Examine how the client responds to this.

Role-play 2 – giving help

Briefing for patient

You have been referred to your local hospital to see the continence nurse advisor. You are very anxious about stress incontinence, which you have experienced since the birth of your last baby two years ago. Although you know your way around the hospital quite well and can find your way to the clinic, you are embarrassed about the problem and therefore have come alone rather than with your partner. You do not speak English, but you have been told an interpreter will be present.

Briefing for nurse

Mrs Janowitz is on your list of patients to see this morning. You are aware she has had stress incontinence during the last two years since the birth of her last baby. You have met her briefly on a previous occasion, and know she does not speak English. You have therefore asked an interpreter to be present. However, there has been some difficulty in finding a person who speaks the same language as Mrs Janowitz; you have not worked with this interpreter before.

As a part of your assessment, you will need to ask Mrs Janowitz questions about her normal pattern of micturition, when she feels she is incontinent, how often, what triggers it off, and so on.

Briefing for interpreter

You are a porter, but have been asked to interpret for the nurse in the clinic this morning. You feel rather annoyed as this will prevent you from getting on with your work, however, you want to do your best to help and have had some experience of interpreting in the past. You arrive early in order to meet the nurse and to arrange your chair between the nurse and the patient so they are facing each other and you can see both of them.

As the interview unfolds, you find many of the questions very embarrassing. You do not know how to deal with this, especially as Mrs Janowitz has a lot to say. You try to summarize rather than to repeat everything.

Debriefing

The purpose of this exercise is to explore the nature of interpreting and to enable students to develop skills in order to work effectively with interpreters. In discussing this role-play, a number of points will emerge. Those relating specifically to this exercise are summarized below.

- The interpreter should be fluent in both the nurse's and the patient's languages. Fluency involves more than accuracy in translating: it also requires the ability to convey idiomatic expressions; non-verbal information; an awareness of cultural norms, and honesty if difficulties in translation arise (Launer, 1978; Bal, 1981).

- Consideration should be given as to whether the patient may be embarrassed by or distrust the interpreter, and whether the interpreter may also feel uncomfortable about certain subjects. For this reason, a stranger may be more acceptable than a family member (Bal, 1981).

- The nurse should ensure that the interpreter is adequately briefed about what is required and the topic to be discussed. The interpreter and the patient may need a little time to introduce themselves before beginning the interview. More time needs to be allowed for the interview itself (Bal, 1981).

- If the nurse and patient sit opposite each other, they may be able to pick up each other's non-verbal cues. Seated in the middle, the interpreter can adopt a neutral position.

- Using a family member as an interpreter may not be acceptable to the patient, especially if it is a child. Children cannot be expected or relied upon to act as fluent interpreters, and if the matter to be discussed is a sensitive one, their involvement may disrupt normal parent–child relationships.

- Staff who are employed in positions other than interpreters may not always feel able to fulfil the role. They may argue it is an 'extra' for which they do not get paid, and that frequent absences from their work, however important, will create friction with their colleagues (Mares et al., 1985).

- In Britain, staff usually have no special training as interpreters or in working with them. This compares markedly with Sweden, where trained interpreters must be provided by law (Watson, 1985).

QUESTIONNAIRE: HEALTH AND ILLNESS

Give each member of the group a copy of the questionnaire below and ask them to answer each question in the spaces provided. Time: 10–15 minutes.

1 *Who makes the decisions in your family?*

   Does each family member have particular responsibilities?

   Is anyone in particular in your family responsible for health matters?

2 *When you are ill, who do you tell?*

   What do you expect this/these persons to do for you?

3 *Think of the last illness you had:*
   – How did you know you were ill?

– How would you describe the symptoms?

– What, in your opinion, caused the illness?

– What, in your opinion, made you well again?

4 *How would you set about visiting your GP?*

During the consultation with your GP do you expect:
– To be asked questions?

– To be given a physical examination?

– To be given a prescription?

ANSWERS

There are no right answers to the questionnaire, but the following points may be useful in discussing each question.

Question 1

Western society and health-care systems reflect the 'cult of individualism' (Benner and Wrubel, 1989), meaning that each person is regarded as autonomous, with a duty to be responsible for him or herself. In this context, the individual can make decisions without reference to others. In reality, however, most people will consult others about important decisions, and the extent to which they do so is both socially and culturally defined.

Hull (1988) found that in Central African societies, illness is a family affair in which the course of treatment is decided by relatives, with elders in particular playing significant roles. The welfare of the children, for example, is very much the responsibility of the grandmother rather than of the natural mother, a concept which differs quite markedly from Western notions about child care.

Question 2

Norbeck and Tilden (1988) state that there is a relationship between informal support-networks and health. Such networks exist in all cultures, but each shapes the behaviours involved. In her study of the concept of care, Leininger (1981) identifies a wide range of behaviours that could be interpreted as caring, for example touch, and that the importance attached to each behaviour varies from one society to another.

Question 3

The social explanation of the nature and cause of disease is often very different from that offered by medical textbooks, and several writers have commented on the interpretations made by different cultures. Cohen (1982) found that the Garifuna (Black Caribbeans of Honduras) recognize a class of illnesses, such as 'mal ojo', which are unknown outside their own society. Wilkinson (1986) found that the Kikuya people, of Thika in Kenya, believe ill-health comes about because of witchcraft; the perpetrator has to be identified in order for the treatment to be completely effective.

In Britain, the inadequacies of the health service provided for members of ethnic minorities can lead to misunderstandings and poor standards of care. Littlewood and Lipsedge (1988), among many others, comment on the high numbers of male Afro-Caribbeans admitted to psychiatric hospitals. Where language barriers exist, the situation is made worse. Wright (1983) describes a survey of GPs in Newcastle in an area where the Pakistani population predominates. The Pakistani women spoke little English and, according to the doctors, often presented with trivial complaints, which were regarded as 'simply a nuisance', but when the language barrier was removed complaints disappeared.

Question 4

Consulting a GP can involve many different things, such as making the appointment; answering questions; having a physical examination if appropriate; possibly being referred to a specialist; receiving a prescription; and so on.

Other, non-Western, systems of medicine do not work on the same principles; their focus is often more holistic than Western health-care systems, with the aim being to treat the whole person. Traditional Thai medicine, for example, has been well established for thousands of years. During the consultation the doctor will ask the patient to describe his symptoms, look in his eyes, note his colour, and take his pulse. The patient is never required to strip off his clothes. Treatment may include herbal remedies and advice about diet and lifestyle. There is no tradition of surgery, since it is not compatible with an holistic approach.

Nolan (1989) describes traditional healers in rural Ireland who are thought to have special gifts or powers, rather than special training. Considering the numbers of people who consult these healers, it is not easy to dismiss such claims. If they were ineffective, few would consult them.

SUMMARY

This chapter has explored a range of everyday activities such as eating and drinking, communication and consulting a doctor. It has demonstrated how consideration of these activities can promote self-awareness as well as insight into cultural differences that exist. In the next chapter this theme is further developed with regard to assessing and planning care.

REFERENCES

Bal, P. (1981) Communicating with non-English speaking patients. *British Medical J.*, 283, 368.

Baxter, C. (1988a) Culture shock. *Nursing Times*, 84 (2), 36–8.

Benner, P. and Wrubel, J. (1989) *The Primacy of Caring*, Addison Wesley, Menlo Park, California.

Central Statistical Office (1991) *Social Trends 21*, HMSO.

Cohen, F. (1982) Transcultural nursing. *Nursing Leadership*, 5 (pt 1), 10–14.

Evers, H. *et al.* (1988) *Community Care Working Papers*, Dept. of Social Medicine, Birmingham Univ.

Fransman, L. (1982) *British Nationality Law and the 1981 Act*, London Fourmat Publishing.

Harrington, B. (1988) A world split open, *Open Mind*, Nov., Encl.

Hull, M. (1988) Child Caring responsibilities in a contemporary Zimbabwean village, conference paper presented at the Anthropology and Nursing Conference, London. Address: Anthropology and Nursing Assoc., Centre for the Study of Primary Care, 384 Commercial Road, London E1 0LR.

Kushnik, L. (1988) Racism, the NHS and the health of black people. *International J. of Health Services*, 18 (3), 457–70.

Launer, J. (1978) Taking medical histories through interpreters, *British Medical J.* Sept. 30, pp. 934–5.

Leininger, M. (1981) Transcultural nursing: its progress and its future. *Nursing and Health Care*, 2 (7), 365–71.

Littlewood, R. and Lipsedge, M. (1988) Psychiatric illness among British Afro-Carribeans. *British Medical J.*, 296, Apr 2, 950–1.

Mares, P., Henley, A. and Baxter, C. (1985) *Health Care in Multiracial Britain*, Health Education Council and National Extension College.

National Assoc. of Health Authorities (1988) Action not words: a strategy to improve health services for black and minority ethnic groups, National Assoc. of Health Authorities.

Nolan, P. (1989) Folk medicine in rural Ireland, *J. of Ethnological Studies*, **27**, 44–56.

Norbeck, J. S. and Tilden, V. P. (1988) International nursing research in social support: theoretical and methodological issues, *J. of Advanced Nursing*, **13**, 173–8.

Watson, P. (1985) Tower of Bable. *Nursing Times*, Dec. 3, pp. 40–1.

Wilkinson, S. (1986) Why there are no accidents in Thika. *Nursing Times*, Apr. 30, pp. 49–51.

Wright, C. M. (1983) Language and communication problems in the Asian community, *J. of the Royal College of General Practitioners*, Feb., pp. 101–4.

FOUR

Assessing and planning transcultural care

Teaching Transcultural Care: A guide for teachers of nursing and health care. Paula McGee. Published in 1992 by Chapman & Hall, London. ISBN 0 412 44080 6. © 1992 Paula McGee

This chapter seeks to develop the knowledge and understanding of transcultural issues gained so far, and to address them within the framework of care provided by the nursing process. It is a continuation of the teaching package, and contains material that can be used either towards the end of the foundation course or during the branch programme. The chapter is structured as follows:

- The issues involved in assessing in the transcultural domain are discussed. Assessment is focused on facilitating personal contact between students and members of local communities in order to learn about values, customs, and beliefs.
- Planning, including examples of care plans that incorporate the principles of transcultural care, is explored.
- Issues involved in evaluating care are described.

ASSESSMENT

Assessment is a crucial activity in nursing. Without a detailed and accurate patient/client assessment, the nurse cannot plan or deliver any form of individual care (Chapman, 1985).

All nurses are expected to be able to assess within the nursing process framework, however, the focus of each assessment will depend on the theoretical framework used. In the transcultural-nursing field, Leininger (1978) defines assessment as a 'systematic appraisal or examination of individuals, groups and communities as to their cultural beliefs, values and practices'. She argues that an assessment should include all aspects of the individual's lifestyle, but also a broad view of the culture in which they live. Thus the cultural value system is important if the nurse is to provide acceptable care that does not offend deeply held beliefs. Similarly, while caring acts are universal, their interpretation and importance vary from one culture to another, and therefore the nurse needs to identify those which are used when planning appropriate intervention.

Since Leininger published her ideas, a number of other nurse theorists have devised cultural assessment tools (Brownlee,

1978; Orque *et al.*, 1983; Gagnon, 1983). The majority of these tools are very detailed, complex, and designed for American health-care situations.

An examination of these assessment tools raises a number of issues. There seems to be little written about their use with individual patients/clients, which is not to say there is no literature on how the principles of transcultural care may be applied. Orque *et al.*, (1983) for example, describe how their assessment tool might be applied to the care of Reza/Latina patients. (Reza/Latina is a term used in American texts to refer to people of, for example, Hispanic, Italian or Latin-American origin.) However, the trend is to focus on groups, and there seems to be a dearth of information on applying specific tools to individual patients/clients.

There is likely to be a strong element of bias in cultural assessment tools. Tuck (1984) draws attention to the possibility of this occurring, especially in the psycho-social domain. She argues that the items listed in any assessment tool must 'be representative of the ethnic/racial patients being assessed'. Examples might include: 'What is the patient's perception of illness, . . . What elements of the dominant culture are health enhancing for this . . . group . . . [and] which are detrimental?'

This is important because the patient/client will probably be assessed by a member of the dominant culture – a phrase which in this context takes on a dual meaning. The nurse might be a member of the majority culture within the society concerned; and health-care professions have their own cultural norms, which tend to predominate in health-care settings (Leininger 1970, 1976, 1978; Hart, 1987). Tuck maintains that this situation creates the possibility of bias and racism not only in the data-collection phase of assessment, but also during the process of interpretation. She recommends that 'interpretation of the data must be done with the knowledge of the specific culture or in collaboration with colleagues from these ethnic/racial groups. Simple intuitive interpretations by nurses of the dominant culture are not valid'.

The concept of assessing 'culture' as an element separate from the psychological, sociological, and other domains is a form of bias in itself, highlighting the idea of culture as a problem created by 'them' – ethnic minority people – who are different from 'us' – the dominant culture. It is incompatible with the philosophy of patient/client-centred care, in which each person is assessed holistically as an individual. Established assessment tools from other theoretical bases can provide relevant data about the cultural domain in a more integrated form (Tripp-Reimer *et al.*, 1984). Moreover, the nurse has to decide whether it is necessary to complete every aspect of the assessment. Given the length and complexity of some cultural-assessment tools, completion could well be a life's work, and of little relevance to the situation in hand.

How, then, can nurses develop the knowledge-base required to assess competently and sensitively within existing frameworks? If the focus of care is individually based, the nurse needs to be educated in working with and listening to individuals before beginning to plan care. In this context, the insistence by several writers on personal contact between nurses and local members of ethnic minority groups becomes very important (Leininger, 1970; Gagnon, 1983; Mattson, 1987). Such contact promotes an awareness of both the differences and the similarities that may exist between two or more cultures; it also encourages the nurse to reappraise her own and professional culture, and facilitates the sensitivity required to provide truly individualized care.

This view is supported by the work of Sands and Hale (Chapter 1), who argue that nurses need to examine their prejudices, apprehensions, and stereotyped attitudes towards economically impoverished clients, and to identify factors that contribute to dehumanized care. Nurses should then be facilitated in learning about local, racially mixed areas through a structured form of personal contact. The knowledge and understanding gained can be used to develop practical strategies in the delivery of individualized care.

Sands' and Hale's approach is deceptively simple, but requires considerable skill on the part of the teacher. Its strength lies in its applicability to all nurses, and therefore it has the greater likelihood of impinging directly on patient care. From the teacher's point of view, the question arises of how best to facilitate such a programme of study. Two approaches are outlined below.

FACILITATING PERSONAL CONTACTS

Educational visits

During the last ten years, the author has frequently taken groups of students on visits to, for example, a Sikh temple. Here, the students had the opportunity to look around; observe a short part of the service; see other facilities such as the school-room; and eat a meal and talk with members of the Sikh community.

Such visits can be very useful as part of a structured programme. Apart from giving a very valuable glimpse of another way of life, it can bring home to students what it means to be a stranger or outsider in a situation where everyone else knows what to do – something that must be experienced by many members of ethnic minority groups whenever they visit a hospital.

Such visits require careful preparation, including:

- An awareness of the broad issues involved in cultural self-awareness, equal opportunities, communication, health, and illness (Chapter 3).
- An introduction to, for example, Sikh beliefs and traditions from a member of the community. This is not to say that all of Sikhism can be condensed into a single lecture, but that students can learn in a positive way by listening to Sikh people talk about what being a Sikh means for them.
- Briefing on,
  – What to wear. In this case, everyone should wear clothes that cover the body as much as possible, including arms and legs, and bring a scarf or hat to cover their hair.
  – What to expect. The students will be asked to leave their shoes at the door. In Sikh temples people sit on the floor, with their feet tucked away from the place where the book of scriptures is placed. Men and women sit in separate

areas. The atmosphere may be less formal than a Christian church, and the Sikh temple is very much a social/ community centre.
– What the students want to know. A list of points to look out for or to ask about is essential. Part of the experience of being the outsider or stranger may be a feeling of being lost and unable to take everything in. Students have reported being overwhelmed at 'being given so much – food, friendship, attention, and not paying for it or being able to give anything in return' (McGee, 1990).

Length of time. Two to three hours' preparation, plus two hours for the visit, and a one-hour debriefing.

Making personal contacts

The author (1990) has described how students can be encouraged to form personal contacts with local members of ethnic minority groups. Over a period of three classroom sessions, students developed a simple questionnaire to help them learn about the way of life within different ethnic groups with particular reference to health care (Table 4.1).

Table 4.1 Extract from class questionnaire

Clothing:	Religious requirements, such as uncut hair? Cultural mores? Getting dressed/undressed – who can help?
Hygiene:	How often does the person wash/bathe? Who may assist them? How do they care for their hair and skin?
Language:	What language(s) are spoken? Who would be accepted as an interpreter?

Once the tool was agreed, each student was given a free choice about which group he or she wished to study. The teacher discussed their choice with each student, and made suggestions about who to contact. Students had to use their own initiative to follow up suggested contacts, visit people, and try to gain information. Despite the difficulties involved, students reported that this encouraged them to utilize a research-based approach, and that they appreciated the opportunity 'to try and find and study objectives and tasks for myself' (McGee, 1990).

It must be acknowledged, however, that some students may find the work difficult, not only because it places great demands on them in terms of using their initiative, but also because their negative attitudes towards other ethnic groups may intrude. Consequently, while the activities above may appear to be very loosely structured, they in fact require considerable planning and supervision. Preparation should include:

- An awareness of the broad issues involved in cultural self-awareness, equal opportunities, communication, health, and illness (Chapter 3), leading into the discussion of knowledge, attitudes, and beliefs about local ethnic minorities.
- It is essential that the teacher has undergone the experience of making personal contacts him or herself, and has developed a sound knowledge-base of the locality, including the different ethnic groups, which can be shared with students.
- Reading and discussion, in order to facilitate the development of a questionnaire by the students, should be encouraged. This is not a rigid list of questions to which the students must adhere, but rather a guide or prompt to assist them and to structure note-taking.
- Plenty of time to undertake the work. A time-lapse of eight to ten weeks between the launch and completion of the work is realistic. Students will need time to form contacts and to get to know people. Regular tutorials or interim feedback sessions will enable the teacher to monitor the progress of individual students, and to provide support as needed.

While many ethnic minority people welcome nurses who undertake this form of study, seeing it as a positive step in improving health care delivery, others may be less enthusiastic. There may be a number of reasons for this. Assimilation into the dominant culture may be seen as a priority, and consequently people may resent any intrusion that reinforces the view that they are different. Others may regard their way of life as a private matter that does not concern anyone else, especially if in the past they have been studied a great deal and are understandably fed up with this. Professionals may be seen as agents of authority and their motives as suspect. Finally, people who have experienced discrimination and racism or have felt dehumanized by the health-care system may not welcome further contact with members of this group. These points are an important part of the regular tutorial work as students begin to experience personal contact with people from ethnic minorities.

- There should be a plenary session in which students share what they have learned and reappraise their original knowledge, attitudes, and beliefs about the ethnic minorities studied. This can then be used as a basis for future sessions on planning care.

PLANNING CARE

The following exercise will enable students to consolidate the material covered in the teaching package and to apply it directly to patient care. The exercise can also be used within the context of teaching nursing theory and exploring its application to clinical practice. Students need to develop ideas about the best way to conduct and set out assessments. Chalmer's (1988) excellent book *Choosing a Model* gives some superb illustrations as to how this can be achieved.

Case study

With particular reference to the concepts of transcultural care, and using a model of nursing, outline the assessment and plan of care you might make for this woman when she is admitted to hospital. Time: 20 minutes.

Mrs Somsri Sawadikul is a Thai who speaks English. She is 62 years old, and a widow. Mrs Sawadikul lives with her married daughter, who gave birth to her first child two months ago. She has been very involved in helping her daughter, and caring for the baby.

During the last year, Mrs Sawadikul has been experiencing difficulties with her bowels – bouts of diarrhoea and bleeding followed by constipation; abdominal discomfort, and feeling generally unwell. She has recently lost weight. She has been very worried about this but felt it was too private a matter to discuss with anyone. Mrs Sawadikul finally went to the doctor with great reluctance. She was deeply shocked to be told she had cancer, and required an operation.

Mrs Sawadikul has been admitted for an abdoperineal excision of rectum. This is her first time in hospital. She is very anxious about the operation – how she will be looked after while she is unable to care for herself and whether she will have to undress.

The following outline assessment and care plan are intended to show how the ideas discussed so far can be applied to direct nursing care using the Roper method of nursing. They contain only the points relevant in providing culturally appropriate care.

Table 4.2 Case study – outline assessment using the Roper model of nursing

Activities of Living (AL)	Assessment of Usual Routine	Actual (A) Potential (P) Problems
Maintaining a safe environment	Khun Somsri feels some things are too private to discuss with other people.	May be reluctant to ask for help. (P)
Communication	Khun Somsri speaks English but may not understand idiom.	Pre- and postoperative teaching may not be understood clearly. (P)
Breathing	No specific points.	

Table 4.2 *Cont.*

Activities of Living (AL)	Assessment of Usual Routine	Actual (A) Potential (P) Problems
Eating and drinking	Khun Somsri probably prefers Thai food.	Supply of Thai food. (A) Advice about diet postoperatively with regard to colostomy. (A)
Eliminating	Khun Somsri normally cares for herself without help from others.	Will feel embarrassed at being cared for by others, especially with regard to catheter care and learning to manage colostomy. (P)
Personal cleansing and dressing	Khun Somsri normally cares for herself.	May feel very embarrassed at being washed, etc. (P) Worried about undressing. (A)
Controlling body temperature	No specific points.	
Mobilizing	No specific points.	
Working and playing	Has been very involved in helping her daughter and caring for her grandchild.	May feel very anxious about how they will cope without her. (P)
Expressing sexuality	No specific points.	
Sleeping	No specific points.	
Dying	Khun Somsri is probably a Buddhist, and may wish to practice her religious beliefs.	

Table 4.3 Case study – outline plan of care using the Roper model of nursing

Problem Related to (AL)	Goal	Nursing Care
Communication Pre- and postoperative teaching may not be understood clearly.	Will be able to communicate effectively. Will be able to demonstrate understanding of teaching.	Use appropriate form of address (i.e. Khun Somsri). Allow plenty of time for conversations and teaching. Avoid colloquial expressions. Ask Khun Somsri to demonstrate/repeat stages to show she has understood.
Eating and drinking Supply of Thai food.	Will receive Thai food, served appropriately.	Find out if there is a member of the family/ friend who can cook for her. Arrange access to ward kitchen if needed. Provide appropriate utensils.
Advice about diet postoperatively	Will receive appropriate advice on diet.	Discuss normal diet with patient and family and dietician (spices and chillies best avoided).
Maintaining safe environment May be reluctant to ask for help.	Will not have an accident while in hospital.	Explain that in the immediate postoperative period she will need help with all her daily functions. Anticipate needs to avoid accidents.

Table 4.3 *Cont.*

Problem Related to (AL)	Goal	Nursing Care
Eliminating Will feel embarrassed about catheter and colostomy.	Will learn to colostomy herself. Patient will not be exposed/distressed.	Demonstrate respect for privacy by not exposing patient or having a lot of people in the room, and by enabling her to do what she can for herself postoperatively. Use video/diagrams to demonstrate colostomy care.
Personal cleansing and dressing Worried about undressing.	Will not be exposed/distressed.	Explain that she will need help in initial postoperative period. Ensure that privacy is respected by not exposing patient, especially during bedbaths and wound dressings.
May feel embarrassed at being washed.		Wash face first and then the rest of the body, ending with the feet. Keep the number of people in the room to a minimum.

EVALUATING TRANSCULTURAL CARE

The question of evaluating transcultural care in practice is as yet untouched, and there is an urgent need for research in this field. In some respects this neglect is not surprising as evaluating care generally receives less attention than the other three stages of the nursing process.

With regard to evaluation and transcultural nursing, there are specific points to be addressed. First of all, how should the evaluation be conducted, and who should carry it out? Goals will form the centrepiece of any evaluation, but determining whether these have been fully achieved can be problematic. The same arguments that Tuck (1984) has pointed out regarding problems of bias in interpreting assessment data can be used for evaluating care.

There is no evidence as far as patients/clients are concerned that transcultural care actually makes any difference; there is, however, some anecdotal evidence that it brings about changes in the attitudes of health-care workers (Stern, 1985; McGee, 1990), and that members of ethnic minority groups welcome their efforts. As one student put it, 'I feel happy and relieved that finally other cultures and my own are being recognized, and something constructive within the system is being done to at last try to cater for other cultures.'

SUMMARY

Direct personal contact between students and members of ethnic minority groups, facilitated by experienced teachers, is an essential part of developing skills in transcultural care. The principles of transcultural care can be applied within the framework of familiar models of nursing and the nursing process. Evaluation of care is a neglected area requiring research, however, evidence suggests that the teaching of transcultural care can be evaluated. This is discussed in the next chapter.

REFERENCES

Brownlee, A. T. (1978) *Community, Culture and Care*, C. V. Mosby, St Louis.

Chalmers, H. (1988) *Choosing a Model*, Edward Arnold.

Chapman, C. (1985) *Theory of Nursing – Practical Application*, Lippincott Nursing Series, Harper and Row.

Gagnon, A. (1983) Transcultural nursing: including it in the curriculum. *Nursing and Health Care*, 4 (3), 127–31.

Hart, L. (1987) A ward of my own in *Social Anthropology of Nursing* (ed. P. Holden), Croom Helm.

Leininger, M. (1970) *Nursing and Anthropology: Two Worlds to Blend*, John Wiley, New York.

Leininger, M. (1976) Two strange health tribes: Gnisrun and Enicidem in the United States, *Human Organisation*, **35** (3), 253–61.

Leininger, M. (1978) *Transcultural Nursing: Concepts, Theories and Practices*, John Wiley, New York.

Mattson, S. (1987) The need for cultural concepts in the nursing curriculum. *J. of Nursing Education*, **26** (5), 206–8.

McGee, P. (1990) The preparation of student nurses for transcultural care settings. Unpub. dissertation. East London Polytechnic.

Orque, M., Bloch, B. and Monrroy, L. (1983) *Ethnic Nursing Care*, C. V. Mosby.

Roper, N., Logan, W. and Tierney, A. (1985) *The elements of nursing*, Churchill Livingstone.

Sands, R. and Hale, S. (1988) Enhancing cultural sensitivity in clinical practice. *J. of the National Black Nurses Association*, **2** (1), 54–63.

Stern, P. (1985) Teaching transcultural nursing in Louisiana from the ground up. *Health Care for Women International*, **6** (1–3), 175–86.

Tripp-Reimer, T., Brink, P. and Saunders, J. (1984) Cultural assessment: content and process. *Nursing Outlook*, **32** (2), 78–82.

Tuck, I. T. (1984) Strategies for integrating African–American culture into transcultural nursing. *J. of Nursing Education*, **23** (6), 261–2.

FIVE

Evaluating the teaching of transcultural care

Teaching Transcultural Care: A guide for teachers of nursing and health care. Paula McGee. Published in 1992 by Chapman & Hall, London. ISBN 0 412 44080 6. © 1992 Paula McGee

Evaluation is a crucial issue in any course if the teacher is to maintain standards and meet the needs of the students. It is of even greater importance when introducing new subject areas into the curriculum. The teacher will need to establish the success or otherwise of the course content; and there may also be a need to justify it to colleagues who are sceptical. Evaluation is also useful in developing a resource-base for colleagues, thus ensuring that transcultural care does not become a 'speciality' taught only by 'experts'.

This chapter addresses three issues with regard to evaluating the teaching of transcultural care: attitude change; academic attainment; and students' perceptions of content. The aim is to explore ideas and possibilities, rather than to provide a blueprint. As in previous chapters, concepts from mainstream education are included alongside those from transcultural nursing literature and research.

THE NATURE OF EVALUATION

There are many different models of evaluation, which may be divided into two groups. The agricultural–botany model (Parlett and Deardon, 1977), which some writers describe as the experimental model, resembles a scientific experiment. The format usually comprises a pretest, following which subjects are either subjected to different conditions/treatment, or entered into a control group. Both are then tested again. The results enable the evaluator to draw conclusions about the efficacy of the treatments/conditions administered.

The illuminative model is concerned with the description and interpretation of events rather than their measurement and prediction (Parlett and Deardon). Here, the aim is to study a teaching programme in a naturalistic way, documenting how it operates, the influences upon it, and the strengths and weaknesses of it as perceived by those involved. The key concepts examined are the instructional system, in which the ideal is compared with the reality, and the learning environment/social context, which will have some unique features.

Illuminative evaluation is not a standard methodological

package, but a general strategy that allows the evaluator to follow a flexible, rather than predetermined, plan (Munro, 1977). It does not preclude elements of the experimental model, but is much broader. As McCormick and James (1983) state, it aims to:

> . . . portray the full complexities of any educational experience . . . it is permissible, indeed desirable, to draw on the whole range of data sources from standardized tests through 'systematic' observation schedules, inventories and pre-coded questionnaires to instructed interview and participant observation. The principal criterion for their selection should be their capacity to inform judgements about a particular activity.

Illuminative evaluation appears to offer the best strategy for evaluating the teaching of transcultural care, especially in the early attempts to introduce it into the curriculum. Its flexible nature allows the teacher to collect data from a variety of sources, and thus reduce the possibility of bias. There are, however, some disadvantages in this approach in that, unless the methods used are carefully structured, the information obtained may appear too subjective (Munro, 1977; Hammersley and Atkinson, 1983).

The flexibility of an illuminative evaluation allows for the use of more than one method – a technique which in research methodology is termed 'triangulation' (Campbell and Fiske, 1959). This is essentially 'the combination of methodologies in the study of the same phenomena' (Denzin, 1989). It allows for both the development of new approaches to a problem, and the emergence of features that would otherwise be overlooked (Jick, 1979).

METHODS OF EVALUATION

Attitude change as a result of teaching transcultural care

Gunter (1988) devised a programme of study for post-qualified nurses with an interest in transcultural care. The focus of the course was a study of Afro-Caribbean culture, and students were required to visit Jamaica for the experience of living and working in another culture. Gunter's main evaluation tool was a before- and-after course measurement of attitude changes using another cultural group (Vietnamese) as a control. While Gunter's students did show more positive attitudes to Jamaican people following the course, student attitudes to the Vietnamese people were much higher both before and after the course. This raises a number of issues; the choice of control group may have been questionable in the post-Vietnam War era; the type of scale used; and whether attitude change was temporary or enduring.

While few teachers will have access to the type of resources enjoyed by Gunter, attitude change would seem to be the most obvious and potent method of evaluating teaching in this field. There is a wide range of attitude scales, and the choice would appear to be straightforward, however, there is a central problem of which attitude to measure. There is a large number of scales measuring attitudes to specific ethnic groups, but considerably fewer that attempt to measure subjects' attitudes to groups other than their own without specifying anyone in particular. In a multiracial society this is a sensitive issue; focusing on attitudes to a particular ethnic group could create unneccessary controversy, alienating both students and others. Even social distance scales that claim to measure attitudes held by the subject towards other groups can prove unsatisfactory. For example, the author (1990) found that the Bogardus Social Distance Scale proved useless in measuring attitude change, and provoked hostility from students.

In addition, individuals frequently say one thing and do another. Berg (1966) demonstrated that attitudes towards people of different ethnic groups can be affected by the setting in which the individual finds him or herself. Subjects who show prejudice on testing may behave otherwise in certain situations, and vice-versa. This might be because certain attitudes are more important to particular personalities than others. In Berg's view, measures such as the Bogardus Social Distance Scale might not measure aspects of attitudes towards ethnic minority people that are central to personality structure.

ACADEMIC ATTAINMENT

Leininger (1984b) clearly saw transcultural care as a post-qualifying speciality in which nurses were prepared at a Masters or Doctoral level. Other writers often do not mention formal assessment strategies in any way. The result is a lack of clarity with regard to what constitutes good practice in the teaching and assessing of transcultural care, especially below the level of Masters degree.

Rowntree (1977) argues that assessment is an important part of any evaluation strategy because it 'reveals to us the most important class of "effects" – the changes brought about in the knowledge and understanding, abilities and attitudes of our students.' On a more cynical note, teachers will recognize that work that is not assessed tends to assume a low priority in the minds of students and, on occasions, of staff.

The author has demonstrated that it is possible to assess students through the medium of a short written assignment (1990). This focused on the student's understanding of the concept of assessment, and the issues each had encountered in assessing one ethnic minority patient/client. The assignment was summative in that it was set at the end of the teaching package, but formative in that detailed written comments were returned to each student by the markers. Sixty-four percent of students achieved the standard required to pass at the first attempt, and the remaining thirty-six percent at the second attempt.

STUDENTS' PERCEPTIONS

Stern (1985) has described how she took 'careful notes on how students and other audiences reacted to what I said and how I said it', using grounded theory methodology. She demonstrated that it was the teachers' attitudes that had the most effect on the students' perceptions of the teaching material. Essentially the concept was one of respect: whether students felt the teacher respected them and invited and utilized their contributions; and whether the teacher made the ideas relevant to their situations, which proved the most effective teaching strategy.

Stern used a form of participant observation (Denzin, 1989) to evaluate the introduction of transcultural care into the curriculum. This requires quite a high level of skill, but has the advantage of potentially yielding detailed accounts of students' reactions to events, as well as the unexpected. The author (1990), for example, found students demonstrating behaviour that could be interpreted as racist.

An alternative approach might be to ask students to complete some form of questionnaire or diary on a regular basis. While there are several predictable difficulties with this approach – the structuring and coding of the questionnaire/diary; the circumstances under which it will be administered – it can yield useful results. The author (1990) found that diaries were helpful in constructing a 'league table' of both the content of a teaching package and the teaching strategies used. Stern (1985) commented that 'clinical logs . . . demonstrated increased sensitivity to other ethnic health beliefs' among graduate students.

SUMMARY

This chapter has explored some of the issues involved in evaluating the teaching of transcultural care. This is a neglected aspect of the literature, and consequently there is no clear yardstick against which to measure good practice. The most useful approach would seem to be an illuminative strategy, using more than one method of evaluation. Participant observation, student diaries, and some form of written assessment can all be included. The advantage of such an approach is that it allows for the unexpected to emerge, and enables the teacher to develop an holistic view of events in the classroom.

REFERENCES

Berg, K. R. (1966) Ethnic attitudes and agreement with a negro person. *J. of Personality and Social Psychology*, 4, 215–20.

Campbell, D. and Fiske, D. (1959) Convergent and discriminant validation by the multitrait–multimethod matrix. *Psychological Bulletin*, 56 (2), 81–105.

Denzin, N. K. (1989) *The Research Act*, Prentice Hall.

Gunter, L. M. (1988) Notes on a method for teaching transcultural nursing, in *Recent Advances in Nursing: Issues in Cross-Cultural Nursing*, (ed. J. M. Morse), Churchill Livingstone.

Hammersley, M. and Atkinson, P. (1983) *Ethnography: Principles in Practice*, Tavistock Publications.

Jick, T. (1979) Mixing qualitative and quantitive methods: triangulation in action. *Administrative Science Quarterly*, **24**, 602–11.

Leininger, M. (ed.) (1984b) Transcultural nursing: an overview. *Nursing Outlook*, **32** (2), 72–3.

McCormick, R. and James, M. (1983) *Curriculum Evaluation in Schools*, Croom Helm.

McGee, P. (1990) The preparation of student nurses for transcultural care settings. (Unpublished dissertation) East London Polytechnic.

Morse, J. (ed.) (1988) *Recent Advances in Nursing: Issues in Cross-Cultural Nursing*, Churchill Livingstone.

Munro, R. G. (1977) *Innovation: Success or Failure?* Hodder and Stoughton.

Parlett, M. and Deardon, G. (1977) *Introduction to Illuminative Evaluation: Studies in Higher Education*, Pacific Soundings Press, CA. Reissued 1981, Society for Research into Higher Education, Univ. of Surrey, Guildford.

Rowntree, D. (1977) *Assessing Students: How Shall We Know Them?* Harper and Row.

Stern, P. (1985) Teaching transcultural nursing in Louisiana from the ground up. *Health Care for Women International*, **6** (1–3), 175–86.

Contact names and addresses

Below is a list of contact names and addresses. It is not exhaustive, but can be used as a basis for discovering what advice and support might exist locally for individuals belonging to a particular religious or ethnic group. For the teacher the contacts will help to develop a network of resources for the teaching of transcultural care.

GENERAL (ORGANIZATIONS NOT AFFILIATED WITH PARTICULAR ETHNIC OR RELIGIOUS GROUPS)

British Red Cross Society

9 Grosvenor Crescent
London SW1

The Red Cross can provide cards which translate a number of everyday terms used in health care situations into a variety of languages. The cards are free.

Local Education Authority

Each authority should have a multicultural support unit that provides advice for teachers in local schools and colleges of further education. Nurse teachers, while not having direct access to this service, can find out about resources and books, and gain advice.

Public Library Service

Some public library services have adapted to provide books and other publications for local ethnic minority groups. Teachers and students could access this service to find out about newspapers and magazines that circulate within a specific group. Alternatively, it may be possible to locate popular novels written by members of other ethnic groups. If these are available in translation, students could use them as a resource.

Commission for Racial Equality

Elliott House
10–12 Allington Street
London SW1E 5EH

The Commission publishes a range of material of use to health-care workers.

British Humanist Association

13 Prince of Wales Terrace
London W8 5PG

National Secular Society

702 Holloway Road
London

Both of these organizations provide advice and support for people who do not profess any religious belief, for example in arranging funerals, and so on.

National Extension College (NEC)

Order Dept.
18 Brooklands Avenue
Cambridge CB2 2HN

The NEC has recently published a booklet *Coming into Hospital*, which is available in Arabic, Bengali, Chinese, Greek, Gujarati, Punjabi, Turkish, Urdu, and Vietnamese. A range of other publications is also available.

The Interfaith Network for the United Kingdom – A handbook
of affiliated organizations

Available from
5–7 Tavistock Place
London WC1H 9SS.

A directory providing contact addresses and organizations of specific religious and inter-faith groups.

ETHNIC (ORGANIZATIONS AFFILIATED WITH SPECIFIC GROUPS)

Afro-Caribbean

The Africa Centre

38 Kings Street
London WC2 8JT

The Africa Centre provides exhibitions, films, plays, school liaison, and other services for those interested in African culture.

Asian

Asian Family Conciliation Service

Princes Chambers, 3rd Floor
Corporation Street
Birmingham B2 4RN

A secular organization offering help, guidance, and support to people with marriage and relationship problems. The service is orientated to the Asian way of life.

Buddhist

The Buddhist Society

58 Ecclestone Square
London SW1 V1PH

The Society aims to make known the principles of Buddhism, and to encourage the study and practice of these.

Chinese

Chinese Community Centre

146 Bromsgrove Street
Birmingham B5 62G

A service providing help and advice for Chinese people, including translation and help with social security matters.

Irish

Federation of Irish Societies

97 Old Lane
Beeston, Lancashire L511 7AQ

An organization which promotes the interests of Irish people living in Britain.

Islam

The Islamic Centre

146 Park Road
London NW8 7RG

The Centre caters for the religious, educational, and social needs of the Moslem community.

Jews

Federation of Jewish Family Services

221 Golders Green Road
London NW11 9DW

The Federation has a training unit for non-Jewish staff employed in homes for the elderly. There is also a large division, Jewish Care, which provides care for elderly Jews, plus a service for those with learning difficulties (Ravenswood) and for children (Norwood). The Federation may be able to help in contacting local Jewish support agencies such as the Jewish Welfare Board, kosher meals-on-wheels, and homes for the aged.

Index